Workaholics Anonymous

Book of Serenity

Weekly Meditations for Recovery

Workaholics Anonymous

Book of Serenity

Weekly Meditations for Recovery

First Edition
Conference Approved 2018

Workaholics Anonymous
World Service Organization

Box 289, Menlo Park, California 94026-0289,
USA
www.workaholics-anonymous.org

ISBN: 978-1-7325768-0-3

Serenity Prayer

*God, grant me the serenity to accept the things
I cannot change,
courage to change the things I can,
and wisdom to know the difference.*

Preface

The Book of Serenity was created to support the important principle of prayer and meditation through the Eleventh Step of Workaholics Anonymous ("W.A."). Once the inspiration came to compile the meditations for the book, a committee was needed to do the task. At the time, W.A. was quickly becoming an international fellowship and it was important to attract a committee that represented as many aspects of that global community as possible.

Because our book would be written by workaholics, we knew we might struggle with ego, perfectionism and impatience. In order to accomplish our task, we would need to make our connection to Higher Power primary and create policies and process that would support our decision-making in a fair and effective way. Our recovery as individuals had to be honored as well. We needed to remember that we had each chosen to be willing channels for W.A. fellowship Higher Power. To support this goal and to protect ourselves and the W.A. process, we decided to require a unanimous decision made by the full Committee each time we voted on any aspect of the book. This protected the process from any one member "taking over" and also allowed Committee members to be fully informed and able to respond to questions from the fellowship. We all worked hard to be good resources for the *Book of Serenity*.

With the Meditation Book Committee in place, the question of how to find meditations became our next focus. Our *Book of Serenity* needed to be written by the W.A. fellowship. We asked the fellowship to write meditations for the book and over 250 meditations were submitted.

One of the most important tasks we had was to honor the themes that emerged through the meditations. We wanted to evolve those themes to a level we knew could help the whole fellowship, honor the intentions of the authors and support the book in becoming a useful tool. We wanted the book to feel fluid, but clear, sensitive and strong. We wanted the book to be a resource for struggles a member might have, a guiding force for change and an easier way to communicate with one's Higher Power. The book could allow people to slip into that place inside them where they could feel their Higher Power and their own serenity and peace.

During the six years of reading, editing and choosing meditations we discussed many ideas about how to format and present each meditation and how to format and edit the book itself. We considered using the Steps as the structure or using the Promises as our guide. We asked about preambles and glossaries and indexes and whether to use the Principles or the attributes. We began to feel a higher energy and insight become our guide and show us how to evolve the book. We realized that in the *Book of Recovery* and *Book of Discovery* we already had the structure for recovery and healing that was needed. What we wanted now was a meditation book that allowed the reader to find their own guidance or theme for healing. It became clear that too many layers (Tools, Steps, Traditions, etc.) began to make the experience feel too guided by program process, and perhaps the member might lose their personal experience of meditation.

When we come to Step Eleven in our program we are at a special place. We have taken the action steps in recovery and done significant work to arrive here. The place of spiritual prayer and meditation is where we can fully open and listen to the guidance of our Higher Power.

As we felt our process come to a close we realized the *Book of Serenity* had shown us how it wanted to evolve and open and soothe us. Always, in recovery, we had worked hard to leave no stone unturned. And through that same recovery we had learned to listen to Higher Power and act from that guidance. The collaboration of the Fellowship of Workaholics Anonymous gave us the *Book of Serenity*.

Appreciation is expressed to each and every W.A. member who submitted their heartfelt meditations to the Literature Committee of the World Service Organization. Many thanks are extended to the Meditation Book Subcommittee for tenderly preparing these meditations for publication. Please continue to submit meditations as we prepare an expanded meditation book that includes 366 entries: one for each day of the year (including leap year). Instructions on the submission process may be found at www.workaholics-anonymous. org.

Cover Art: The beautiful cover of the *Book of Serenity* was originally created for the cover of the first Workaholics Anonymous book. In 2004, World Service Board members suggested that three elements be incorporated into the cover: 1) A symbol of slow movement (a snail was requested); 2) a symbol of time; and 3) the concept of spaciousness. What resulted was: 1) the overall image of a nautilus shell (home to the sea snail); 2) the sun, moon and stars (symbols of time) incorporated in the central circle of the nautilus, with stars placed on the circle of the sun in analog clock position; and 3) spaciousness denoted in the central circle – looking out to the galaxies, beyond, and the swirls of the nautilus shell as they expand outward. Warm appreciation is extended to the artist, a W.A. member.

A huge, sincere, "Thank you" is extended to all who participated in this process. And without the Higher Power of Workaholics Anonymous, this *Book of Serenity* would never have come to pass.

Foreword

One of the resources suggested by the Workaholics Anonymous program is meditation. Meditation offers us opportunities to take quiet moments to be still, reflect on our experience, and remind ourselves of the foundations of our recovery. The meditations in this book offer food for thought as you take this time to reflect. They are based on submissions from W.A. members from throughout the fellowship. May they lead you to greater serenity and sanity.

Suggested uses for this book:

- Personal reflection and journaling
- Inspiration during daily self-care breaks
- Reading aloud during group meetings

The quotation under the title of each meditation is taken from Conference-approved Workaholics Anonymous literature.

Weekly Meditations for Recovery

God's Soft Voice

Before accepting any new commitments,
I ask for guidance from a Higher Power.

In the everyday throng of voices and demands, God's soft voice is like a whisper. To hear it, I need to pause, feel my breath and become quiet.

God knows about my daily difficulty of making choices. God also knows which work project I should tackle and which one is not for me to do. God knows if it's better for me to stop and do nothing. If I hear and follow God's whispering, nothing bad can happen to me.

I create silent moments to ask God
if I'm on the right path.

Ego Boost or Serenity?

Even when offered the best, I say "no" if I need rest.

I enjoy my work so much that when an opportunity to use my skills comes along, I get excited. Even with no room in my schedule, I can feel drawn to the new project like an addict to a drug. I quickly see myself as the perfect person to take it on. My adrenaline and my ego get a boost, but soon my serenity takes a dive.

Thanks to the Program, I know I'm not indispensable. Even if I'm the best person for the job, my peace of mind requires me to say no sometimes. I no longer want to endure the stress and strain of overdoing. If sensations of stress arise when I think about this new project, I pay attention. They can be my Higher Power's nudge, signaling me that saying no is the best thing I can do for myself and for the project.

Saying no can be a way of saying yes to sanity.

Step Three

Made a decision to turn our will and our lives over to the care of God as we understood God.

My first reaction when I read Step Three was tremendous relief: "God will take care. I can let go of my enormous willpower, constantly driving me here and there, wanting this, wanting that – always wanting more."

The next thoughts that dashed in: "Oh, goodness! How will I manage to turn my will and my life over? How will I do this properly? How can I get it all right?"

Much later it dawned on me that I have to do nothing more than *make the decision.* I can simply turn inward, let silence fall in the inner chamber of my heart, and there, as in the contemplative silence of a chapel, *make the decision.* I hear my voice saying softly and firmly: "Yes, God, I decide to turn my will and my life over to your care."

Nothing more is needed.

Today I make the decision.

Pacing

We rest before we get tired.

When I first heard these words about the recovery tool of Rest, they baffled me. How would I know when I was going to get tired before it actually happened? What if I ended up resting nearly all the time, just in case? I'd never know if it had been necessary or how near I had been to getting tired. And surely I didn't deserve to rest until I had finished everything there was to do.

After some time of practicing this tool, I have become much more in tune with my body and my energy levels. The balanced rhythm of activity and rest, followed by more activity and rest, has become as natural to me as breathing in and out, in and out.

Thanks to my Higher Power, I live by a tool that I could not understand with my own reasoning.

I am grateful for the promises coming true in my life.

A Relationship with God and Myself

*My relationship with a Higher Power
has given me my life back.*

Over a very short period of time, the W.A. principles and tools have seeped into my life and changed it. With the almost daily help of a sponsor, I am beginning to see how work and activity addiction blocks me from God. I let others know me. I read the W.A. literature and attend meetings. I pray and meditate daily. As a result, I now find myself delighting in the desire to slow down, breathe deeply and enjoy a calm pace.

W.A. teaches me how to be comfortable in my own skin. Establishing a relationship with God enables me to get to know my true self. What an abundant gift!

**I connect with myself and
my Higher Power daily.**

Sanity and Insanity

We are able to change our thoughts to healthier ones.

I am an addict. That means I do things that have a harmful effect on me. I delude myself about this and keep doing the same things over and over again. I suffer as a result of this behavior and tend to blame God and the world for it. My attitude becomes ingratitude. That's insanity.

Recovery started when I became more and more honest with myself. I recognized the harmful essence of my addiction and admitted it. I let go and let God. I shared my feelings with others and new things happened in my life. It seemed like a miracle to me. I began counting the good things in my days and felt good. My attitude changed into gratitude. That was sanity.

Gratitude is the attitude of sanity.

Step Eleven

We find we need the light and love of our contact with our Higher Power.

I have decided that my daily time for prayer and meditation is the most important part of my day. It is the first thing I do each morning. Some days I have less time for it than others, but I am grateful I have been able to do it regularly. Some religious traditions talk about bringing the first fruits of material possessions to God. I also want to bring the first fruits of my time to God and spend time with God first thing in the morning.

Conscious contact with God is my number one priority every day.

Affirmation Giggles

Time is my friend.

When I first heard the affirmation "Time is my friend" read out loud at a meeting, I burst into laughter. The concept was so foreign it seemed ludicrous, the exact opposite of my experience.

Yet time is my friend. What is my life except the time gifted to me for the years I walk this earth? Affirming this truth puts a little wedge of distance and doubt between me and the disease that wants to run my life and ruin everything.

Best of all, the phrase still makes me giggle. A space opens in my chest. My shoulders relax. My jaw releases its clench. It's the light touch of truth providing relief against the heavy hand of disease. My disease has no sense of humor. Laughter immediately nudges me out of the stress of stinking thinking and into recovery – if only for a moment. This moment of time in recovery is indeed an especially good friend. It invites me back to play again.

**I have all the time I need to do
what is mine to do.**

Serving

We ask for help and reach out to help others.

When a W.A. member showed me how to write an abstinence plan for myself, my recovery started in earnest. These moments of service by another W.A. member gave me the foundation on which my recovery is built.

I now gain a lot by passing on what I have learned to other workaholics. I relive the feeling of first being shown the program myself, with extra gratitude, connection and joy.

Of course, to enable my Higher Power to give me these experiences, I need to be present and under-scheduled. I need to have my own example of recovery and serenity to share, motivating me to stay close to my program.

**Higher Power, I am grateful for
Step Twelve.**

Openheartedness

We freely admit our weaknesses and mistakes.

I used to believe that the world was an ungenerous place and that the people in it were even less generous in their attitudes towards me.

I projected an image of competence and knowledge as armor, and I used dishonesty about my weaknesses as a wall to hide behind. I never gave the world a chance to view me with warmth, acceptance and compassion.

Yes, there are people in the world who judge others to escape seeing their own faults. I suspect nearly all humans do this. Yet I now recognize that most of the time people are much more loving and accepting than I previously believed.

Admitting my weaknesses and mistakes allows me to experience being loved for who I truly am.

Breaking Illusions

There will be enough time, love and money.

I am discovering I am enough. I am whole. I am part of something much bigger that is full of love.

I've spent so many years trying to be perfect, caught up in the illusion of who I need to be in the world to be acceptable, safe and at peace. I've experienced so much struggle and pain chasing this illusion, performing and achieving at all costs. Then, one day, the illusion was smashed and I was lost. I wondered, "Who am I without my qualifications, power, and sense of organizational belonging? Who am I, and how can I be of service to the world?"

My Higher Power assured me: "You are a part of me, we are whole. You are love. Together we can restore balance. You will have all you need."

I am not my work.

Let Go and Let God

Letting our Higher Power guide us requires giving up control.

I love to walk labyrinths. Sometimes I pause to pray at each turn. Sometimes I just look at the surroundings. One of the things I like best is just watching my steps without giving any attention to where I am or where I'm going.

For me this is a real change. In the past I always wanted to know where I was and to feel certain that I was safe and in control. In a labyrinth, often the closer it appears you are to the center, the farther away you actually are. And then, when the end seems the farthest distance away from you, you are closer than you think. It's just like life. I've plotted my way, felt lost, hesitated, turned around, tried to get back and then found myself right where I needed to be.

I take the steps and trust that Higher Power will take me where I need to go.

Program Calls

*We reach out to stay in contact
with other W.A. members between meetings.*

When I first came to W.A., my phone weighed 300 pounds in my mind. I had a great deal of trouble picking it up. I didn't want to disturb my fellow workaholics – I knew they were busy. Besides, I didn't think my problems were worth troubling another person.

Over time, W.A. friends began to call me. I learned that program calls are a gift to the person who receives the call as much as to the person who reaches out. When I make a call or take a call, the conversation always helps my recovery.

**Today I know that help
is only a phone call away.**

Living Like a Cat

Let go and flow.

When my cat needs to rest, he rests. He does not spend an hour tidying up first or cramming in just a little more work to "earn" his nap. When my cat feels like playing, he embraces his inner kitten and really goes for it, unconcerned about being called stupid or lazy. He attends to his self-care without hesitation, never pausing to check his to-do list first. My cat is present for every moment of his life; he does not waste hours meticulously planning the future or analyzing the past.

My cat is happy, joyous and free.

I am not a cat. I'm a human being with responsibilities and complex feelings – and a full-fledged addiction. But through my willingness to rely on a Higher Power and to work the W.A. Twelve Steps gently and lovingly, I'm learning to look after myself as well as my cat looks after himself.

Recovery from workaholism offers me the chance for a new life every day.

Loving Acceptance

I don't try to grow.
I accept myself as I am, and I grow
automatically.

Again and again I get into workaholic conditions.
Of course – I am a workaholic! But often I don't
want to admit it. I also have the illusion that
the Program will make me recover overnight.
I condemn myself for my "failure." I want my
recovery to be perfect.

My sponsor told me I could understand sobriety
in workaholism as the capacity to perceive when
I am acting in a workaholic mode and then stop
doing so.

Just for today I want to treat myself lovingly.
When my inner child stumbles and falls, I will
comfort and encourage this innocent, learning
side of myself to stand up and try again.

Falling is not failure if I pick myself up.

Hastiness

Space out activities to avoid becoming spaced out.

At times, I want so badly to get everything done that I forget to pace myself or to be realistic about how much time each job takes. Most often, this hastiness is born out of fatigue and frustration. When I'm depleted, I tend to feel rushed.

In W.A., I'm learning to take time for myself first. I can sit in a chair for a while or take a deep breath. If these simple activities seem impossible, I try to be gentle with myself and exercise caution before adding to an already frantic schedule.

When I do plan some open time to relax, it helps if I begin by praying for the patience and willingness to leave that time open and to take good care of myself.

Just for today, I will leave some open space in my schedule to unwind, breathe and relax my body.

Serenity Underneath

*We try to live each moment with serenity,
joy and gratitude.*

One night as I was walking my dog, feeling unloved by my wife, sorry for myself and inadequate, an idea hit me: Perhaps serenity is not something to be attained but is already here. Perhaps the muddy waters in my life are my own creation, and underneath all that roiling is the bedrock of serenity, unchanged and unmoving.

I realized that I was afraid to let go of the thrill, the grasping and the victim/star status and just be a guy with countless blessings walking a dog. I feared that underneath it all, there might be *nothing*. I decided to reach beyond these fears and trust that only the deep peace of serenity awaited me. I went for it – I chose to still the waters. And there it was. It only lasted for a few minutes, but it was powerful and true. I felt the possibility of new life.

**I surrender to my Higher Power, allowing
myself to drop into serenity.**

Glow Flowly

The slower I go, the faster I grow.

When I first heard the word "flowly" in a W.A. meeting, I had to laugh. Just for fun, I added the word "glow" in front of it, and I became fond of that phrase!

Then I spotted a very large, heavy concrete garden turtle in an import shop. That turtle spoke to my heart, "Take me home!" I purchased her and with much help got her home, where she sits on my hearth. Her name is "Glow Flowly." To me, she symbolizes gentleness, leisureliness and connection to a Higher Power. Her head is tilted upwards and her feet are still, reminding me to be calm and still and to ask Higher Power for guidance.

**I'm taking my time and having
a good time doing it.**

19

Anonymity

Anonymity is the spiritual foundation of all our traditions.

Soon after finding W.A., I came to realize that a major drive for my workaholism was my need for recognition. Since childhood I had felt invisible. In order to be seen, I worked extremely hard at school and on the job. Anonymity in the Program was a challenge for me. I asked myself, "How will people know my value if I remain anonymous?" Over time, I realized that the group already valued, accepted and supported me. Anonymity allowed me to strip away external labels and find myself. This was the beginning of true sobriety.

The deep transformation of accepting myself as *just me*, rather than someone's boss or caregiver or parent, eventually spread to other parts of my life. I was no longer interested in "networking," but very interested in connecting to others. I became much more friendly, warm and accepting to family, friends and co-workers.

Today I will take a risk to meet others as another human being – not using titles or achievements as my calling card.

20

Sun Rising

A will of steel had gotten us through long workdays and sleepless nights.

Each morning, the sun rises. I never noticed the sunrise when I was in the depths of my workaholism. It seemed banal, a given, something the universe owed to me. I only used the sunrise to mark the time of my work hours. I was all powerful. I could ignore the laws of nature, including the laws of my body. All that mattered was getting the job done, and done *perfectly*. The very fibers of my being craved the prestige and satisfaction that flowed from my work, which I did at all hours of the day and night. I was sick. Very sick.

Eventually, I became willing to turn my will and my life over to the care of a Higher Power, whose love for me knows no bounds. Now I rise with the sun, and when it is nighttime, I sleep peacefully. For that I am ever grateful.

**I rise each day to shine brightly
as I serve my Higher Power.**

21

Well Done

Good enough is still good.

When I first heard the slogan "Good enough is good," I cringed. How could *good enough* be good? It wasn't an *A+*, or even an *A*, for that matter. I recalled my father never being happy with all my *A*'s and one *B;* that wasn't *good enough.* His way of thinking stuck with me.

But when I sat with the slogan, something in me relaxed. Good enough *is* good. The pressure is off. I don't have to be perfect, or even the best speaker or the best organizer. I don't have to expend myself completely on my work tasks. I can do a good job today without adrenaline and have enough energy to be present to the rest of my life after 5 p.m. Even though I never heard it from my father, I can say "Well done" to myself for doing a good enough job.

**I am grateful for Program slogans
that remind me how to recover.**

22

Focus

Be here now.

One of the gifts of W.A. is learning how to focus. Doing one task at a time, praying for the ability to concentrate, using a daily plan and under-scheduling are all helpful tools.

My overly busy mind can cause me to lose focus and miss moments of being fully present. If I give my full attention to this very moment, I could be noticing sensations of an early morning breeze or sounds coming through the window. I may hear the rattling of paper, rolling wheels of a cart or a song on the radio.

The Eleventh Step reminds me that my life has a spiritual purpose expressed in this moment. Guidance for living this purpose comes when I focus on the now and become quiet enough to hear. I may even find it's time to rest. If so, I take that rest, finding my energy and focus renewed when I return to my work.

**Every moment is a gift from
my Higher Power.**

23

Meditation

Sought through prayer and meditation to improve our conscious contact with God as we understood God.

After a busy day of being intensely focused and feeling rushed and pressured, meditation can seem impossible. How can I meditate with my mind racing like this?

I sit anyway and open up my mind. As my awareness comes into the present moment and broadens out to my Higher Power's world that surrounds me, I need nothing else. Just the awareness of my Higher Power's presence is enough to bring me peace.

My breathing slows. The spikes of focus smooth out to become a part of the greater landscape of my existence. My presence in the world has a depth and vibrancy that it didn't have before.

Any time is a good time to meditate.

24

Affirmations for Workaholics

My Higher Power wants me to realize my vision of joyful work and a balanced life.

On days when I feel stressed, challenged or in need of some extra inspiration, I say a quick prayer asking for an affirmation for the day. Glancing through the list of affirmations in the *Book of Recovery*, I let myself be guided to a place on the page where I feel the "click" of intuition as I read a certain affirmation. Now I have an affirmation for the day to help meet my needs for support and encouragement!

I write down this affirmation and keep it nearby, using it throughout the day to inspire my thoughts and actions. Doing so helps me to feel more peaceful and cared for, make better decisions and keep myself on the recovery path. My stress is reduced and my life is more satisfying.

I trust my Higher Power to give me whatever I need at the right time.

25

Time

There was a lack of reality with time.

Before W.A., I used to say that I needed thirty-six-hour days and twelve-day weeks in order to accomplish everything I needed and wanted to do. There was never, *ever* enough time.

The literature of Workaholics Anonymous told me that I could become "a friend to time." I had no idea what that meant. I found it baffling and confusing at first.

Today, as I use W.A.'s principles and tools, I rarely think of time as either my friend or my enemy. The clock is neither my master nor my slave. Time is only a product of the human perspective.

Workaholics Anonymous is teaching me that there is enough time, money and love and that everything can wait except love. Maybe, after all, I'm becoming a friend to time.

**Sanity is doing only what I have time
to do with serenity.**

26

Fearless Inventory

*Made a searching and fearless moral
inventory of ourselves.*

What does it mean that my inventory is fearless?

Is it that, having done Steps One, Two, and Three,
I am feeling no fear, particularly about this step?

Maybe this is the case for some. For others, the
thought of taking inventory of our shortcomings
can be a source of trepidation. Even if I do
experience some degree of fear, however, I do not
have to let it affect my inventory. I can still look
at the truth squarely and steadily, committing it
to paper.

Maybe, just as when I was small and checked for
monsters under the bed, I might find there was
nothing to be scared of after all.

**I welcome my fear as a sign
of my willingness to grow.**

27

Exercising My Faith

We began to recover by gradually removing our irrational thinking and habits with the help of a Higher Power.

When I obsess about a challenging person or situation, what I often need is a boost of faith. At these times, taking the Third Step can help me let go and let Higher Power. When verbal prayer does not bring relief, I write my prayer to seek the spiritual help I need.

First I jot down what troubles me. Then I write, "I am making a decision to turn this over to my Higher Power, who…," adding a few thoughts about how I've been helped in the past and who my Higher Power is to me at this time.

After letting go of my concern, I jot a brief description of what I feel and think now, compared to when I was upset and obsessing. Turning my problem over to my Higher Power is exercising my faith muscle, and I can see the results of that strengthening immediately and over time.

I can make a decision at any time to turn my will and my life over to my Higher Power.

28

Integrity

I am more effective when I am more selective.

I used to believe that the only way to gain the respect of my superiors was to defy them. This led to acts of self-sabotage and a string of gap years. I was both frantically busy and barely employed.

Now my Higher Power guides me toward both acceptable behavior and awareness of my needs. I am able to act with integrity – even when I say no.

One Friday, my employer was clamoring for me to work weekend hours. Instead of making excuses or demanding to be paid triple-time, I consulted my Higher Power, drew a temporal boundary, and let the work wait until Monday. I enjoyed a weekend of relaxation, self-care, exercise and socializing. On Monday, my Higher Power provided me the strength to perform the work still awaiting me. No surprise, as the work – and the weekend – were both within the flow of **G**ood **O**rderly **D**irection.

I make choices today that are respectful of myself and others.

29

Progress

*I am gentle with my efforts, knowing that my
new way of living
requires much practice.*

Sometimes, I really enjoy the fruits of my recovery
from workaholism –feeling present in the moment,
approaching life with grace and humility, feeling
warmly connected to my Higher Power and
others. Yet, a few days or weeks later, I find myself
feeling rushed, insecure and overwhelmed again.

I might wonder if I have made any progress at all!

When I go to the sea to watch the tide come in, I
see the waves surging in to fill the beach, and then
retreat back out to sea. By being patient and staying
a while, I might see that, during the rhythmic ebb
and flow, the tide has been imperceptibly but
surely moving in toward the shore.

**When I focus on recovery in the midst of
the ebb and flow of life, I draw closer to
serenity.**

30

Relaxing

***When we feel energy building up,
we stop and reconnect with a Higher Power.***

Today I want to spend some time relaxing and enjoying the silence with my Higher Power. I want to quiet my crazy thoughts and allow peace and joy to flood my mind and body. I take a deep breath and exhale all the stress, anxiety, control and "must do's" flooding my mind. I can put all this strained thinking aside for a while today and then go back later to take on my chosen tasks with serenity. I know there is recovery in a quiet mind.

When I focus on my anxiety and fear, my life becomes tumultuous and exhausting. When I let harmony and peace take their place today, I can relax.

**With a relaxed mind, I allow love and joy
into my life, and divine order is restored.**

31

Patience

The slower I go, the faster I grow.

Often in my workaholism, I am impatient, stressed out, irritated and anxious. I have a difficult time allowing circumstances to unfold at a natural pace. I am irritated when others don't work at my pace or in the way I want things done. The more anxious I feel, the more irritable I become. I begin to spin out of control and become completely overwhelmed. This is never good for my mind, body or spirit. Usually the task I am trying to accomplish suffers as well.

Today I will begin to cultivate patience. I know that everything unfolds in God's perfect order and timing. My job is to relax into it. I will try to silence the voices in my mind that tell me I must do everything at once, do things faster or do more than I planned.

I cultivate patience and allow solutions to come naturally.

32

Stop

Be here now.

I wake up in the morning and mentally go through my daily "to do" list. So many important things that I can't miss! I'm late. I'm late and I'm tired. Last night I had to finish that unavoidable piece of work. Really I didn't have much time to sleep.

Well...

I stop. I stop the hurry. I stop the list.

I get up and open my bedroom window. I look outside and greet the new day the Universe is giving me. I thank the Universe.

I smile. I breathe. I live. I'm free.

When I start by stopping, I can make sane choices for my day.

33

Step Twelve

*We tried to carry this message to
workaholics, and to practice these principles
in all our affairs.*

How can I carry the message of recovery? I do
it through sponsorship, sharing in meetings,
outreach to the media and professional groups
and serving in our W.A. fellowship.

I also find myself carrying the message in
unexpected ways. Maybe a friend asks me, with a
mix of hope and desperation, if it is true that there
is a program of recovery for people who work too
much. Maybe a family member finally reaches
rock bottom with compulsive doing and asks for
help.

At these times, practicing the principles of
recovery in all my affairs becomes essential. I can
tell people about the tools, Steps and meetings all
I like, but if I am rushed and adrenalized, what I
say will not ring true. I demonstrate the gifts of
recovery by repeated behavior over time.

**As I go about my day with serenity and
presence, I may be carrying the message to
someone who still suffers.**

34

Comparing

I'm perfect just the way I am.

One thing that drives my workaholism is making comparisons: This colleague works more hours than I do, that person does more service, another accomplishes more. I feel less than them and work extra hard, trying to keep up.

Comparing personal qualities also diminishes my joy. I suffer from envy over the co-worker who communicates with relaxed ease or the friend who loves to be around other people.

Trying to match others' abilities is like trying to wear their shoes. It's uncomfortable and I'm not going to get very far.

I feel more at ease and work less compulsively as I examine and honor my own strengths and limits: What pattern of work and rest brings about my best work? What form of service allows my Higher Power to be expressed most fully through me? What form of social interaction leaves me feeling most alive and connected?

Higher Power, help me to care for and nourish the precious work of creation you have made in me.

35

Action Planning

We put on paper what we intend to do each day.

My daily plan is a tool for honesty and recovery. I complete it during my prayer time. I have been given this day by God, and I want to commit to using it well.

How different from the tyrannical "to do" lists that I endlessly made in the depths of my disease! They would contain far too many tasks to fit into a day, and very few items on the list were going to be any fun.

Now, I give priority to relationships – with God, others and myself – and to what I can do to carry the message of Twelve Step recovery. My action plan also includes the daily tasks necessary for sane, orderly living, being self-supporting and having some fun.

When I can share my action planning with another person, so much the better for my sense of reality and self-honesty.

Today I create my action plan as I pray to God for a balanced and spacious life.

36

Acceptance

We learn to want what we have rather than be concerned with having what we want.

There is no way I can control the world around me, even though I may want to. On the contrary, happiness comes to me when I let go and flow with life as it is, harmoniously.

My Higher Power knows better than I do, and I realize my true serenity comes from the acceptance of all that is around me and within me, including my shortcomings. When I stop trying to force things, better things come about.

I have more energy when I accept what is.

37

Learning to Play

The more I play, the more my Higher Power works.

I once took part in a day of play for adults. One activity was to pair up with another person and spend half an hour together in "make-believe" play. My partner was comfortable with playing, and before long we were engaging in a wonderful "child-like" dream. My reaction to this play time was so strong I was literally shaking from the intensity of the experience. I wondered if I had ever experienced such pure joy.

Only years later did I recognize that I had an addiction to working compulsively. Work was my escape, since I didn't know how to play and have fun. After a year in recovery, I am now thoroughly enjoying brief moments that feel like play. I am confident that, with continuing recovery, I will increase my ability to open up to the powerful healing that fun and play offer.

I make plans to play and have fun every day.

38

Slow Speech

The slower I go, the faster I grow.

One sure sign of my workaholism is when I speak rapidly. I know my adrenaline is in full flow. I am not really speaking to connect with someone but to make sure I'm heard. I'm afraid if I slow down, others will stop listening.

One of my bottom lines has become speaking slowly. My communication then becomes an experience of being in mindful relationship with the listeners rather than a mad dash to get everything said.

Slow speech also tends to slow my breathing and my heartbeat, leaving me relaxed.

I speak in an easy rhythm, with no rush.

39

Have a Good Time

Enjoyment of the process becomes our criteria.

Working hard used to be my badge of honor. I liked to impress people with how much I had to struggle to accomplish what I did. If the deadline was short – even better, "impossible" – I would take on a project with zeal. Praise was often my reward, and I relished an inflated sense of self-worth from demanding so much of myself to reach a goal.

Now, when asked to do the impossible, I say no. Also when I start to feel stressed while working on something, I stop, take a breath and ask myself, "How can I have a good time doing this?" Usually a smile emerges and I start singing or dancing to lighten my outlook. I stop pushing and start playing.

**I look for ways to have fun while
I'm getting things done.**

40

Easy Does It

The less I struggle, the more open I am to inspiration.

In the disease, I forced solutions and inflicted my will on others. This demanding approach to life produced only hatred, rebellion and retaliation. The results I was trying to reach would seldom materialize.

In recovery, I try to work effortlessly and with ease. I let other people do their thing and reap their own positive or negative consequences. I surrender people, places, institutions and processes to God and try not to have expectations. I remember, "Easy does it."

I do what God tells me.

41

Courage to Say No

Grant me the courage to change the things I can.

My workaholism, my do-it-all-ism, flourished under an umbrella of codependency. I believed that acceptance by others plus my own self-worth depended on saying *yes* to every request, no matter how overcommitted I already was.

In recovery, the Serenity Prayer seeped through the cracks of my restless facade of activity, and living the program ignited a spark of courage. I began to take time before responding, saying, "Let me think about that and I'll get back to you." By the next morning I usually knew the right answer. Then I was able to deliver my *no* to the person with a one-sentence response, such as: "My plate is pretty full right now" or "This doesn't feel like a good fit."

Saying no was hard the first few times, but that spark of courage has grown into a resilient confidence in committing myself to a healthy balance of saying yes and no.

Saying no is a gift I give to others from my recovering self.

42

One Day at a Time

We are granted only a daily reprieve.

As an active workaholic, my time horizon was never twenty-four hours. I projected my planning five or ten years into the future. Focusing way ahead like that allowed me to escape the daily responsibilities of getting adequate sleep, nutrition, exercise and time off from work for personal pursuits.

Today, I realize that all I have is a daily reprieve. I don't know if I will be here tomorrow, let alone next year or ten years from now. I realize the insanity of running my life today based on what might happen in an uncertain future over which I have no control. Now, when I wake up in the morning, I breathe, relax, smile and say, "I'm still alive!" I am grateful that I made it to another day. I make an action plan just for the next twenty-four hours, and I follow it to the best of my ability.

**I trust that my Higher Power
keeps me alive today for a good reason.**

43

Making Friends with Time

We under-schedule to allow more time than we think we need for a task or trip, providing a comfortable margin to accommodate the unexpected.

From a very young age, I had the habit of rushing *and* of being late. Each time I was late, panic and guilt created intense waves of mental and physical turmoil.

I desperately wanted to be on time and would figure out the best time to leave, then add extra time. But when it came time to go, I would discover "just one more thing" that I felt compelled to do. I thought I could cheat timetables, connection times, traffic and time itself. It was exhausting.

In W.A., I have come to realize the extreme harm of adrenalizing. The body keeps score. Now, if I hear myself using the phrase "I'll just…," I often catch myself and ask, "Do I really need to do it now?" or "Is there enough time to do it in a calm and fully present way?" If the answer is no, I am learning to leave the task for another time.

To avoid adrenalizing, I schedule in buffer time and do tasks peacefully.

44

Nurture

I fuel myself differently these days.

The principle of nurture guides me throughout each day. I extend compassion to my body with all its complexities. I breathe in life and love. I feel, express, explore and then let go of hurt and anger. I nourish my body with healthy food, fresh air, time in nature and frequent laughter.

Today I give myself the whole-hearted nurture of love that I so desperately yearned for, yet was denied. I trust that nurture will also come to me as love from my Higher Power and others in recovery, and love will heal.

Today I will nurture myself physically, emotionally and spiritually with grace and lightness. I will take time to be still. In this quiet state, I will listen to my body whispering its needs. I will gently tend to them, as a mother tends to her baby, with love, compassion and gentleness.

Listening to and loving myself is nurturing and life-giving.

45

Recovery from Activity Addiction

*We can also be workaholic in hobbies,
fitness, housework, volunteering or in trying
to save the world.*

My workaholic rock bottom came when I was limiting my paid work to forty hours per week, yet spending endless hours on recovery. Due to this over-scheduled life, I grew more tense and detached from my feelings. I would add in another meditation group or meeting or concert, trying to bring to my life more peace or fun or whatever I needed.

What I needed more than anything was space to process, rest and just be.

For workaholics, letting go of what seem to be "good" activities can be painful. At first, guilt or profound grief may arise as I step away from doing what is dear to my heart.

The joy comes, however, when I experience the richness of a spacious life. I am able to be fully present and alive in my fun activities. I find true healing as I work my Program. I experience the power of grace manifesting in the service that I do.

**I make space in my life to experience the
presence of my Higher Power.**

46

From Scarcity to Abundance

Fears that there won't be enough time, money or love leave us.

Prior to W.A. recovery, I lived in a universe of scarcity invented by my own mind. I was convinced that there could never be enough time, money, resources, energy, encouragement, love or approval to achieve my goals and thereby wrest happiness and satisfaction from an unkind world. I had to grab what I needed through sheer effort and willpower. The cycle of stress and adrenaline dependency that resulted took me to my rock bottom.

Working the steps of W.A. has slowly allowed me to have faith that following God's healthy plan in my life will provide for my needs. I have noticed how well things work out when I stop using force to make up for the perceived shortage of time, money and love. All that I need to live peacefully in recovery is brought to me through prayer.

Today I will train my muscle of faith to expect abundance.

47

Self-Care

I love myself, no matter what.

Driving myself into the ground is the opposite of self-care. The same is true when I punish myself for not living up to my sky-high expectations or for making a mistake. I no longer want to abuse myself like this.

W.A. has taught me how to love, respect, value and nurture myself. It has been a steep learning curve, but I have gotten back in touch with my feelings. When feeling tired, instead of berating myself for being a "lightweight," I rest. When thirsty, instead of "forging on," I stop and take a drink. When bewildered, instead of running in circles, I call a friend in W.A. I am learning to meet my needs.

Old habits sometimes kick in, but self-care is gradually becoming more habitual than self-neglect. As I show more kindness to myself, I also show more love to others. I feel happier and my self-esteem blossoms.

When I nurture myself and treat myself with love, I start to believe I'm lovable.

48

Step Two

Came to believe that a Power greater than ourselves could restore us to sanity.

I find enormous comfort and relief in remembering this step. I need to remind myself many times each day that this Power exists – an infinite Power which can heal my soul of all its wounds, great and small. For me, it is a Power of infinite strength and infinite tenderness, mighty enough to move mountains, gentle and generous enough to respond to my childlike hurts. Relying on this Power restores my hope, humor and tranquility.

**I find refuge in my Higher Power.
It is my garden, my sanctuary, my home.**

49

Pleasure as a Spiritual Priority

*We allow ourselves to enjoy
the present moment.*

I was taught growing up that life is hard and filled with suffering. "You'd better pull your weight." "Put your shoulder to the grindstone." "Pull yourself up by your bootstraps." So, I pushed and pulled and measured my success by how much I accomplished, how much I impressed others and how far ahead I got.

In W.A., I learned that I can never get enough points on my "scorecard" to feel entitled to rest. I came to see that stopping to smell the roses is the whole point of everything. If I miss the joy along the way, who cares what gets done?

Nurturing pleasure is a spiritual practice and a way of life – one that prioritizes happiness and joy, one that sustains me as it nourishes me. In W.A., I am learning how to value living each moment fully, slowly, easefully.

**In W.A., how I get there takes precedence
over where I'm going.**

50

Service

**_Service to others has helped me
to return to W.A., time and again._**

I've spent much of my life striving to get praise,
money and power in order to feel good enough,
powerful, even exceptional. I was trying to get all
that from other people. What I was really grasping
for was a sense of self.

Today I turn my thoughts to my Higher Power
and practice seeing through God's eyes. I shift my
agenda for the day from what I can get and how
I can get it to how I can _be_ and _serve_. I consider
what gifts I can offer today. A smile, some kind
words or full attention to a worthwhile project –
everything I do can be an act of service.

By shifting my focus to what I can give, my purpose
becomes to serve God. I find peace, contentment
and fulfillment. My life is rich beyond my dreams.

**Today I turn my thoughts from
"What can I get?"
to "What could I give?"**

51

Step Four

As we name our attitudes and write about our patterns, both helpful and unhelpful, we begin to understand ourselves better.

The questions in the Workaholics Anonymous *Book of Recovery* gave me a great starting point for the fact-finding and fact-facing process of Step Four. My sponsor provided a sounding board and reality check. What discoveries – and none of them to be feared!

The writing and naming process distilled and clarified the confusion of my workaholic story. Like a face emerging from a block of wood under the carver's chisel, a three-dimensional image of myself emerged, not the chaotic cartoon character I had taken myself to be. This person had some real assets and some real liabilities.

For the first time I could see the physical and psychological forces that had acted on me in the flow of life. I saw where I swam against the tide and where I went with the flow. I saw how I influenced that stream and my fellow swimmers for good and ill.

I have the courage to look at the habits of mind that have driven my actions.

52

Powerlessness

Recovery from workaholism is not a cure, but a lifelong process.

I might come into W.A. looking for a simple cure. I think I can go to some meetings, work some steps, find a balance that is right for my life and get rid of my workaholism.

Instead, I find that recovery from work and activity addiction requires constant awareness and loving attention. Even when I do achieve a balance in my life that brings me serenity for a while, life soon enough disturbs my equilibrium and brings home once more the reality of my powerlessness.

Again and again I have to take inventory, hand my life over and humbly ask for help from others and my Higher Power. Over time, as I work my program, my perfectionistic need to "always get things right" diminishes.

As I lighten the grip of perfectionism, I receive the blessing of constant growth and aliveness.

I embrace the miracle of imperfect recovery.

Appendices

The Twelve Steps of Workaholics Anonymous

1. We admitted we were powerless over work – that our lives had become unmanageable.

2. Came to believe that a Power greater than ourselves could restore us to sanity.

3. Made a decision to turn our will and our lives over to the care of God *as we understood God.*

4. Made a searching and fearless inventory of ourselves.

5. Admitted to God, to ourselves, and to another human being the exact nature of our wrongs.

6. Became entirely ready to have God remove all these defects of character.

7. Humbly asked God to remove our shortcomings.

8. Made a list of all persons we had harmed, and became willing to make amends to them all.

9. Made direct amends to such people wherever possible, except when to do so would injure them or others.

10. Continued to take personal inventory and when we were wrong admitted it.

11. Sought through prayer and meditation to improve our conscious contact with God *as we understood God,* praying only for God's will for us and power to carry that out.

12. Having had a spiritual awakening as a result of these Steps, we tried to carry this message to workaholics, and to practice these principles in all our affairs.

The Twelve Traditions
of Workaholics Anonymous

1. Our common welfare should come first; personal recovery depends upon W.A. unity.

2. For our group purpose there is but one ultimate authority – a loving God as expressed in our group conscience. Our leaders are but trusted servants; they do not govern.

3. The only requirement for W.A. membership is a desire to stop working compulsively.

4. Each group should be autonomous except in matters affecting other groups or W.A. as a whole.

5. Each group has but one primary purpose – to carry its message to the workaholic who still suffers.

6. A W.A. group ought never endorse, finance or lend the W.A. name to any related facility or outside enterprise, lest problems of money, property, and prestige divert us from our primary purpose.

7. Every W.A. group ought to be fully self-supporting, declining outside contributions.

8. W.A. should remain forever nonprofessional, but our service centers may employ special workers.

9. W.A., as such, ought never be organized; but we may create service boards or committees directly responsible to those they serve.

10. W.A. has no opinion on outside issues; hence the W.A. name ought never be drawn into public controversy.

11. Our public relations policy is based on attraction rather than promotion; we need always maintain personal anonymity at the level of press, radio, and films.

12. Anonymity is the spiritual foundation of all our traditions, ever reminding us to place principles before personalities.

Index of Titles

Index of Topics

We welcome your comments and suggestions for the revision of this book as well as for future literature:

Workaholics Anonymous World Service Organization
P.O. Box 289
Menlo Park, California 94026-0289
USA

Telephone: (510) 273-9253
Email: wso@workaholics-anonymous.org
Website: www.workaholics-anonymous.org